I0426670

Photos by http://all-free-download.com/free-photos/download

https://www.dreamstime.com

ISBN 978-1-387-36092-5

Disclaimer

We have used research to conclude the accuracy of these suggestions. **REMEMBER THAT THIS IS A REFERENCE VOLUME ONLY, AND NOT A MEDICAL MANUAL.**

You may choose to seek professional help first. Hopefully these suggestions will inform decisions you make about your future health. Charles Paul Jeffries assumes no responsibilities or liability for injuries, damages, or losses incurred during use of or as a result of this information.

While herbal research is in its infancy, and a lot is still unknown, there have been herbal remedies that have similar effects as pharmaceutical products. This is why we always suggest that you check with your physician before you use them.

Herbs recommended in this book are generally regarded as safe (GRAS).

Natural Holistic Remedies

Guide for helping you heal yourselves naturally with safer alternatives to conventional medicine.

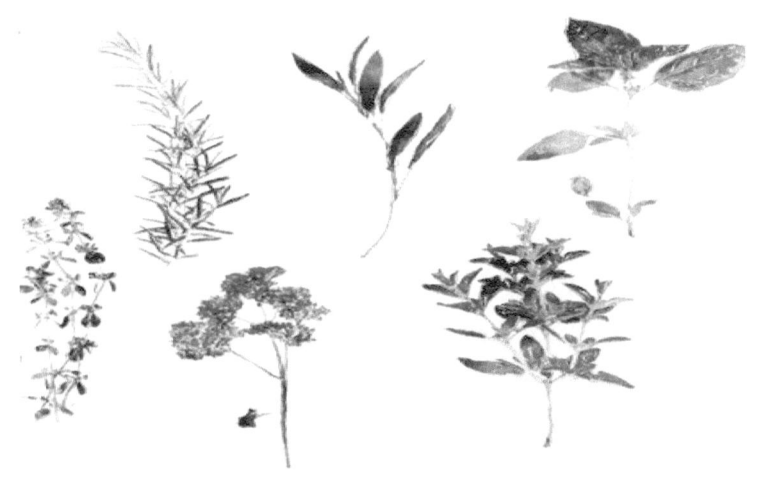

By
Charles Paul Jeffries
BS, MS, Holistic Remedies Certification

Introduction

This book is for those who have decided to finally take control of their health and eliminate the annoying recurrences which have plagued their well-being for years. This is the time that you expand your knowledge of what good health is all about and take an active yet informed role in learning what works for you and your system. While it is well known that today's modern medicines are derivatives of natural plants and herbs which God has blessed us with, few realize that these chemical compounds are inorganic and are often not readily absorbed by our bodies thus causing harmful residual effects. Just listen to the side effects of almost any drug commercial and you will see what I mean.

Contrary to this is the fact that natural herbs are for the most part well absorbed by our bodies and while they might not work as quickly as convention medicines, they usually have little to no side effects.

Take the time to examine the herbs I have listed and the myriad of uses which they portend as well as the herbal teas which have helped so many over the years. You will find yourself embarking on an adventure of self-healing, increased energy, and improved clarity of thought. I wish you "All The Best" as you strive to take control of your future good health.

Table of Contents

Introduction	4
Natural Holistic Remedies	7
Handy List of Herb Teas	20
Rosemary Tea	23
Red Clover	24
Spearmint	25
Peppermint	26
Yarrow	27
Plantain	28
Marshmallow	29
Licorice	30
Lemon Balm	31
Valerian	32
Turmeric	33
Thyme	34
Elder	35
Ginger	36
Echinacea	37
Chamomile	38
Burdock	39
Calendula	40
Alternative Heroes	41
Herbal Contraindications	57
Index	66

Natural Holistic Remedies

I believe my journey towards holistic treatments and theories began when I was just a child. Whenever we would drop our candy on the ground we would pick it up, blow on it, and then say, "Well, you have to eat dirt before you die." Where this childhood logic came from I have no idea, but it helped me set the stage for my curiosity about plants and soil and the role they play in my life.

I remember planting watermelon seeds and watching them grow until my brother ran over them with his bicycle. I remember planting peach seeds and could hardly wait for the seven years I was told it would take to bear fruit. I enjoyed tending to our flower garden and pruning our rose bush and trees. I would pick fruit from our backyard trees, pick greens, snap beans and shuck corn. My father would always tell me that you couldn't eat better than fresh veggies straight from the farm and I always looked forward to eating them.

It wasn't until I reached adulthood that I began to pay attention to the value of herbs and the many benefits they provide. So I jumped at the chance to learn more and develop my knowledge of its many uses.

Throughout history, every culture has used herbs for medical treatments. The early colonists were no exception and brought with them a thorough knowledge of herbal treatments. Exchanges between early colonists and Native Americans promoted the use of local and European herbal remedies. Natives had extensive knowledge of the healing power of herbs which they shared with early settlers.

"When the slave became sick we most time had the best of care take of us. Maser let our old mammy doctor us and she used herbs from the woods such as Cami weeds, peach tree leaves, red oak bark for fever and chills and malaria or things that way that the white doctor could not cure. Yes, our old Negro mammy was one of the best doctors in the world with her herb teas. When she gives you some tea made from herbs you could just bet it would sure do you good." By John Mosley, born 1851 in Texas, "African American Slave Medicine" book.

I feel like recognition and integration of modern holistic medicine to the medical field in general has been a blessing of immeasurable proportions. When I think of the barbaric methods used in ancient times to heal patients which usually ended in horrific pain and then death, I'm awful glad to be alive today.

The genius of holistic medicine is that it takes the whole person into account while working in unison with conventional medicine and different forms of alternative therapies to reach its goals. It proposes that if one aspect of a person's life is out of order that it affects the entire system. They believe that mental, spiritual and physical well-being along with love, laughter and individualistic treatment is the key to optimal health. They explore the entire person to find out who they are as a person. Integrative medicine refers to the use of all types of therapies.

It may include prescription medication, surgery, acupuncture, aromatherapy, mental health counseling, herbal medicine and perhaps yoga. It seeks to treat the whole person instead of a disease, with well-being of the mind and body. It compliments established modes of treatments not replace them. In addition, we still may use regular home remedies even after we see a conventional doctor.

I'm excited that I have learned that herbs are nature's remedy and were placed on this earth by our almighty Creator.

There is an herb for every disease that a human can suffer from. Pioneers grew and exchanged herbs with other cultures for medicine, beauty products and food items. However, the Egyptians were noted as the first people to experiment with herbs and bring about the art of herbology and it was in the middle-ages when herbs were first used in rituals.

It is good to be reminded that the use of herbs is the oldest medical science and therefore one of mankind's oldest forms of healing. I realize that all through our history and even to this day that much has been written about them and continues to be written. It was fascinating to learn that herbs act on our blood and all life processes including the nervous system, therefore they are capable of bringing the body into harmony and balance. Herbs are considered food for the body. They are valuable sources of natural medicine, vitamins and minerals that have a remarkable history of curative effects when used in the proper way. Every plant on this earth has a purpose. Every part of this earth has herbs that provide a service to man or animal. The herbs that are useful for a certain ailment usually contain vitamins and minerals that are also helpful in that particular problem or concern.

All drugs that are extracted in some way from a plant will not benefit the human body in the same way that herbs alone will. Also, I know some of the effects that real herbs and their constituents have on our bodies so I feel that I can try several of them for ailments since they're natural and side effects are minimal. When it comes to chemical medicines, the drug does not contain the entire plant in its natural state, with the natural components and concentrations as they are found in nature. I have learned that chemical drugs are not the answer and never will be. Every drug has some possible side effect. These side effects are increased even greater if a person is taking more than one drug.

Herbs, when used properly, are usually safe and do not leave built up residue in the system to then produce side effects. Nature's herbal remedies can quickly relieve and have a curative value for many ailments. I wish I had this knowledge a long time ago. It would've saved me a lot of money and suffering. Everyone can benefit from using herbs, but the best results will be realized when the body is clean and free from accumulated mucus and toxins. Mucus and toxins are expelled through the skin, nose, mouth, stomach, lungs, kidneys, and colon. Once the body starts the eliminative cleansing the herb will be able to perform its desired tasks even more effectively.

Because of integrative health options, today's health conscious public is now realizing, by consulting with medical doctors and natural health specialists that herbs can bring all around better living through the attainment of good health. Integrative health gives people a choice to choose to go to a doctor for symptom relief or to go to a natural health care doctor for total relief from the same symptom. Conventional methods may be faster but natural relief is safer without side effects and can prevent the need for constant prescriptions and reliance on chemicals. Other modalities such as yoga, acupuncture, massages, therapy sessions, chiropractors and aromatherapy can assist with balancing and healing the body. Integrative health is very important when it comes to taking control of your health care options. Integrative medicine takes into account all dimensions of the individual: mind, body and spirit. Most important is that it empowers patients with new choices and promotes preventative care. For holistic doctors, understanding the client's social domain such as their home life, place of employment, social activities or the environment that surrounds them is a great way to produce the best outcome and care for that person.

Athletes are finding that certain herbs give added stamina and strength. Herbs are helping thousands control weight and keep in shape. As a beauty aid they are far surpassing any of the concoctions of today. Students are finding that herbs enhance their alertness and mental capacity.

Despite the criticism of herbal medicine among mainstream medical professionals, it is wise to remember that many common drugs we use today were derived from plant-based sources. These are just a few examples of why it's important to consider the advantages and disadvantages of herbal treatments.

When integrative health is part of the treatment plan, it's great to know that the choice is there to choose chemical treatment over natural medicines and other homeopathic treatments. Most herbal medicines are well tolerated by patients with fewer unintended consequences than pharmaceutical drugs. Herbs typically have fewer side effects than traditional medicine, and may be safer to use over time. They tend to be more effective for long-standing health complaints that don't respond well to traditional medicine. This is where integrative health is very important. Another advantage to herbal medicine is cost.

Herbs costs much less than prescription medications. Research, testing, and marketing add considerably to the costs of prescription medicines. Herbs tend to be inexpensive compared to drugs. Another advantage to herbal medicines are their availability. Herbs are available without a prescription. You can grow some simple herbs, such as peppermint and chamomile at home. In some parts of the world, herbs may be the only treatment available to the majority of people. I think a course in learning how to grow, harvest and use your own natural products should be taught in high schools and colleges.

Herbs are not without disadvantages, and herbal medicine is not appropriate in all situations. I learned a lot by referring to other herbal books that these are a few of the disadvantages to consider:

- I do realize that there are times when using herbs may be inappropriate: Modern medicine treats sudden and serious illnesses and accidents much more effectively than herbal or alternative treatments. An herbalist would not be able to treat serious trauma, such as a broken leg or a heart attack as effectively as a conventional doctor using modern diagnostic tests, surgery, and drugs.

- Another disadvantage of herbal medicine is the very real risks of doing yourself harm through self-dosing with herbs. While you can argue that the same thing can happen with medications, such as accidentally overdosing on cold remedies, many herbs do not come with instructions or package inserts. There's a very real risk of overdose. That's why taking courses is valuable for improving or maintaining optimum health.

- Harvesting herbs must be done with care, from the time of year to the type of soil used can make a huge difference as to the herb crops you produce. Harvesting is a delicate process. Because one slight mistake such as the wrong soil, too much water or sun can make for a bad crop. A great takeaway is knowing that harvest times are critical and harvest times are not the same for all herbs. Storage and processing are also critical and so is the location where the herb is grown. Herbs that are plentiful in certain locations show that the land is suitable for future harvests of that herb.

- I learned that you must also be careful of what herbs you pick if you're not familiar with them. It's best to harvest them yourself or know the description and properties of the herb to avoid a very real risk of poisoning and making yourself and others sick.

- The knowledge of herbs is valuable because herbal treatments can interact with medications. Nearly all herbs come with some warning, and many, like the herbs used for anxiety such as Valerian and St. John's Wort, can interact with prescription medication like antidepressants. It's important to discuss your medications and herbal supplements with your doctor to avoid dangerous interactions.

- I learned that since herbal products are not tightly regulated, consumers also run the risk of buying inferior quality herbs. The quality of herbal products may vary among batches, brands or manufacturers. This can make it much more difficult to prescribe the proper dose of an herb. Growing and harvesting your own herbs by far is the way to go.

People should be aware of the benefits as well as the precautions involved in taking these natural remedies. Herbal medicine is a part of homeopathy, which is an alternative system of healing that uses very small doses of like substances to relieve specific symptoms like giving a flu shot for the flu yet homeopathy is based on the idea that the body can heal itself. Hippocrates called it the "like cures like" theory. Back in the day, even the Egyptians used homeopathy to cure their ills. However, herbs were a power aid in healing and treating skin issues. According to what I learned, even the Egyptian Queen Cleopatra was very fond of using herbs in her beauty products and aromatherapy.

Studying herbs has been one of the smartest things I could have done to improve my physical and mental health. The knowledge that I have gained about alternative medical practices and solutions has expanded my perceptions and left me feeling empowered and confident enough to take control of my decisions concerning good health.

I have learned so much about herbs that I had already heard of, and even more about herbs that I never knew existed. I learned that every plant on this planet has a particular use and purpose. Even the Bible teaches us that, so I think that it's up to us to seek out the knowledge of these herbs which God has provided for optimal good health.

What has been most fascinating about my herb discoveries has been the incredible usages of each herb. One herb that nearly everyone is familiar with is peppermint. While most of us are well aware of its use in candy, toothpaste, teas and balms, it also offers relief from headaches, nausea, skin irritations, flatulence, diarrhea, menstrual cramps and other health problems. It can also soothe pains, relieve cough symptoms and speed up the digestion process. Not only is it rich in vitamin A and C, it can also cure stress and mental fatigue. You can also make peppermint tincture to apply topically for muscle sores, indigestion, heartburn and even make peppermint soup.

So many of these herbs have similar multiple uses that the average person would not know if they didn't take the time to research or if they were not exposed to this knowledge. Herbs can be made into soups, teas, tinctures, essential oil, incense, hair dyes, shampoo, foot scrub, even salads. I've created a handy list that is just a sampling of the healthy herbs that you can research to improve your health:

Handy List of Healthy Herbs

Herbs for Blood Pressure

- Hawthorn
- Garlic
- Nettle

Bad Cholesterol

- Hawthorn
- Ginger
- Garlic
- Red Clover
- Licorice

Indigestion/Stomach Aches

- Basil
- Chamomile
- Calendula
- Burdock
- Thyme
- Marshmallow
- Lemon Balm

Flu/Colds

- Elder
- Echinacea
- Garlic
- Yarrow
- Marshmallow
- Licorice
- Rosemary

Skin Conditions

- Echinacea
- Aloe Vera
- Lavender

Wounds

- Echinacea
- Basil
- Calendula

- Turmeric
- Thyme
- Peppermint
- Marshmallow

- Garlic
- Lavender
- Yarrow
- Turmeric
- Plantain

Cleanse Blood/Arteries

- Hawthorne
- Burdock
- Red Clover

Muscle Pain

- Nettle
- St. John's Wort
- Rosemary
- Plantain

Immune System

- Echinacea
- Elder

Anxiety/Stress

- Dandelion
- Chamomile
- Lavender
- Valerian
- Lemon Balm
- Spearmint
- Sage
- Peppermint

I have begun to incorporate my new found knowledge of herbs to fight my muscle pain and my arthritis. I created an all-natural pain salve containing Shea butter, cocoa butter, lavender, coconut oil, cayenne, calendula, beeswax, olive oil, eucalyptus, arnica and curcumin. Not only have I experienced significant personal relief, but I have shared this formula with several of my friends and each of them have benefited from this product. I have also developed a natural shaving bar which contains clay, and an anti-aging cream.

I am so pleased with the knowledge that I have gained about herbs and so thankful to be able to share with others and enhance their lives along with mine.

I've also included a list of herbal teas and recipes to assist with some of our most common ailments.

Rosemary Tea

Soothes a worried mind, aids meditation and yoga practice, improves concentration, prevents memory loss, helps fatigue and colds.

Ingredients

1 – 2 sprigs of fresh Rosemary

1 – 2 cups cold water

Tea pot

Natural sweetener (honey or Stevia)

Instructions

Put the water in the teapot and bring to a boil. Add rosemary sprigs to the water and turn off the fire and let the rosemary steep for 3 minutes or more. Add sweetener to counteract the bitter taste.

Red Clover Tea

Used to treat hot flashes and menopausal complications. Has blood cleansing properties, helps lower cholesterol. Relieves stress.

Ingredients

1 cup of red clover blossoms.

A 36 oz jar

36 oz. water

Tea kettle

Peppermint or sage to enhance the flavor (optional)

Instructions

Place blossoms in a the jar.

Put water into the tea kettle and bring to a boil.

Pour the hot water into the jar full of blossoms.

Cover jar with the lid and let sit for about ten hours.

Optional: Add peppermint or sage to enhance flavor and potency.

Spearmint Tea

Kills bad breath, indigestion, nausea, gas, diarrhea, stress and headaches, removes excess body hair in women.

Ingredients

A handful of spearmint leaves

4 cups of cold water

Tea pot

Strainer

Lemon juice (fresh)

Raw honey

Instructions

Put the water in the teapot and let it heat. Take the handful of spearmint leaves and crush them to release the flavor and then add to the heated water.

Let the water come to a boil for 1 minute and then remove the pot from the heat and let steep for 10 – 15 minutes.

Strain into a glass container or tea cup to separate the crushed spearmint leaves from tea.

Add honey or lemon as desired.

Peppermint Tea

Gives relief from headaches, nausea, skin irritations, flatulence, diarrhea and menstrual cramps. Speeds up digestion.

Ingredients

A handful of peppermint leaves

4 cups of cold water

Tea kettle

Strainer

Natural sugar like honey or Stevia

Instructions

Shred the peppermint leaves roughly into small pieces.

Put a cup of water into the kettle and bring to a boil.

Place the shredded peppermint leaves into a steel tea ball or a steel infuser.

Add the tea ball or infuser to the kettle and steep for 10 minutes. Consume tea when it is lukewarm.

For best results, avoid refined sugars. Use honey or Stevia.

Yarrow Tea

Used as a compress to close open wounds. As a tea, rids PMS, cramps, bloating, flatulence, cleanse kidney and urinary tracts, help with circulation.

Ingredients

1 cup of Yarrow

6 cups of cold water

Tea pot

Strainer

Lemon juice (fresh)

Raw honey

Instructions

Bring the 6 cups of water to a boil.

Add the Yarrow and let steep for 5 minutes or more. When the concoction reaches a honey colored tone, strain in a large 70 oz. jar or container and let cool.

Add lemon and honey.

Note: To make the compress, crush the yarrow separately and boil ¼ cup in ½ cup of water, strain and dab on wound a couple of times per day. To use as a poultice, grind herb and put the herb oils directly on the affected area.

Plantain Tea

Treats mouth sores, bronchitis and tuberculosis. As a poultice, plantain alone helps heal wounds and inflammation. Plantain also helps to relieve and heal sore throats.

Ingredients

1/4 cup of Plantain leaves

1/4 Peppermint leaves

Instructions

Shred the peppermint leaves roughly into small pieces.

Put a cup of water into the kettle and bring to a boil.

Place the shredded peppermint leaves into a steel tea ball or a steel infuser.

Add the tea ball or infuser to the kettle and steep for 10 minutes. Consume tea when it is lukewarm.

For best results, avoid refined sugars. Use honey or Stevia.

Note: To make the poultice, crush the plantain separately and apply directly to the wound or boil ½ cup in water, strain and dab on wound a couple of times per day.

Marshmallow Tea

Treats bladder infection, improves gum health, reduces toothaches, soothes nervous tension.

Ingredients

1/4 cup of Marshmallow leaves and roots

1 cup of water

Tea pot

Tea ball

Cinnamon

Vanilla

Instructions

Cut up roots and leaves with a pair of kitchen scissors.

Heat the cup of water in a tea pot, bring to a boil and then pour into a cup. Place the marshmallow leaves and roots in a steel tea ball and place it into the tea pot.

Let steep for 10 minutes. Stir the ball and shake gently to get the maximum extraction of the herb.

Add a few dashes of cinnamon or vanilla for flavor.

Consume lukewarm before it thickens up.

To treat gum or tooth issues, dab the solution on the tooth or gums, swish your mouth and **DO NOT** rinse. For other issues, drink an entire cup at a warm or luke warm temperature.

Licorice Tea

Treats ulcers, colds, constipation, cholesterol issues, minimizes and removes the build up and depositing of arterial plaque, alleviates menstrual cramps, adrenal fatigue and leaky gut issues.

Ingredients

1 teaspoon of Licorice root

36 oz of water

Tea ball

Peppermint leaf or one drop of peppermint oil

Dash of cinnamon

Instructions

Shred one teaspoon of licorice root and put into the tea ball.

Put water into the kettle and bring to a boil.

Add tea ball, peppermint and cinnamon to boiling water.

Remove from stove and let steep for 10 – 15 minutes.

Drink a maximum of 3 lukewarm cups per day.

Lemon Balm Tea

Great source of relaxation. This tea contains lots of antioxidant properties that boosts good health, and treats ailments such as herpes sores, headaches and even treats insect bites.

Ingredients

½ cup lemon balm leaves

Tea ball

2 cups of water

Honey

Instructions

Heat 2 cups of water in a tea kettle.

Grind up the lemon balm leaves and put them into the tea ball.

Before water starts to boil, remove it from the stove and add the tea ball to the water.

Let steep for 10 minutes. Pour a cup and add honey to taste.

Valerian Tea

Remedy for insomnia, anxiety and nervousness. Dubbed as "the poor man's valium". Also good for muscle pain, joint aches, hot flashes and menopause symptoms

Ingredients

1 teaspoon of Valerian root

Tea kettle and 8 oz of tap water to sterilize the tea kettle

Tea pot

Strainer

8 oz of filtered water

Raw honey or milk (optional)

Instructions

Use tap water to boil and sterilize the tea kettle.

After kettle comes to a boil, pour the tap water out and add the 8 oz. of filtered water and bring it to a boil.

Put the valerian root into the clean tea pot and pour the hot filtered kettle water over the valerian root.

Let steep for 15 minutes.

Strain into a cup and add honey or milk if desired.

Tumeric Tea

Great for relieving inflammation and pain. Tumeric is also a cooking spice that adds great taste to foods. Helps relieve arthritis pain, detoxifies the liver, improves digestion and helps to relieve stress. Good for overall health maintenance and healing.

Ingredients

Instructions

1/4 cup grated tumeric root or one tablespoon of ground turmeric

2 tbsp. of grated ginger root or powder

2 cups of water

Fresh lemon juice

Raw honey

Cheese cloth and or strainer.

Heat 2 cups of water in a tea kettle.

Add the turmeric and ginger to the water and boil for 5 minutes and then let steep for 10 minutes.

Strain using a strainer for the root or use a cheese cloth to strain the powdered herb.

Pour a cup and add lemon and honey to taste.

Thyme Tea

Great for treating coughs and colds. Contains antioxidants, vitamins and minerals that aids in treating the flu and improving intestinal integrity.

Ingredients

2 tablespoon of fresh time leaves or dried thyme

2 cups water

Tea kettle

Tea ball

Lemon juice

Raw honey

Instructions

Bring 2 cups of water to a boil in the tea kettle.

Finely chop 2 tablespoons of fresh thyme.

Put the chopped or dried thyme in a tea ball and add it to the boiling water.

Turn fire off and let steep for 10 minutes.

Add lemon juice and honey per cup to taste.

Elder or Elderberry Tea

The elder herb fights the flu, colds, sore throats, boosts the immune system and also helps to lower cholesterol and improve vision

Ingredients

Instructions

1 ½ tablespoon of dried elderberry powder

1 ½ cup of water

Lemon slice

Honey

In the tea kettle, add the elderberry and water and bring to a boil. After it boils for 1 minute, remove from heat and let it simmer for 5 – 10 minutes.

Pour into a cup by straining with a cheese cloth and add the lemon slice by squeezing it and putting the slice into the cup of tea.

Add honey or brown sugar to taste.

Ginger Tea

Power herb that helps to fight inflammation and pain, digestive issues, lowers cholesterol and helps with motion sickness and nausea. Great powerhouse for fighting the flu.

Ingredients

4 – 6 slices of fresh ginger

2 cups of water

1 lemon

Honey or Stevia

Tea kettle

Tea pot

Instructions

To make the best and the potent ginger tea, make sure that your ginger root is fresh and plump.

While boiling 2 cups of water in your kettle, peel and slice or finely chop your ginger and put the ginger in your tea pot.

After the water starts boiling, remove it from the heat and pour it over the ginger that's in the tea POT.

Let sit for 5 minutes and then add the honey and lemon to taste.

Echinacea Tea

This powerhouse herb fights colds and flus, ear infections and helps to heal wounds and skin infections when used as a poultice or compress .

Ingredients

Instructions

2 cups boiling water

Tea kettle

Tea pot

2 teaspoon of dried echinacea flowers

1/2 teaspoon of fresh ginger or ½ tsp of powdered ginger

Cheese cloth

Lemon juice from ½ of a lemon

1-2 teaspoons honey

In the tea kettle boil the 2 cups of water.

While the water is heating, place the echinacea and ginger into a tea pot.

After the water has boiled, pour it on top of the echinacea and ginger in the tea pot and let sit for 10 minutes.

Pour into a cup by straining with a cheese cloth and add the lemon juice and honey to taste.

For wounds or skin infections, to use as a compress, place tea soaked cloth directly on affected spot. In this case, do not use the honey or lemon.

As a poultice, grind the herb and place directly on affected area so that the herb oils can go directly into the wound.

Chamomile Tea

Great herbal sleep aid. Good for stomach issues, digestive aid, stops diarrhea and great for aromatherapy sessions.

Ingredients

2 -3 tsp of freshly picked or dried chamomile leave blossoms

1 cup of water

Honey or Stevia

Lemon

Tea pot

Tea ball

Cheese cloth

Instructions

Put the chamomile into the tea ball.

If using a strainer, put the chamomile directly into the tea pot.

After the cup of water has boiled, pour it over the chamomile leaves in the tea pot or add the tea ball to the tea pot and let it simmer for 5 minutes.

Remove the tea ball and pour tea into a cup. Or, use the cheese cloth to strain the tea into the cup.

Add the honey and lemon to taste.

For aromatherapy, add dried flowers to a dish and let the aroma fill the air.

Burdock Tea

This herb is a natural blood cleanser, diuretic used to flush waste and toxins. Also helps to repair skin issues by flushing toxins from the body.

Ingredients

Instructions

2 tablespoon of dried burdock root

3 cups of water

Stainless steel pot with a lid

Kitchen knife

Chop the burdock root until you have 2 full tablespoons.

Add the burdock root to the pot and cover with 3 cups of water.

Bring to a boil for 1 minute and then turn the heat on low and let simmer for 30 minutes.

Drink 2 – 3 cups per day?

Calendula Tea

The wound healer. Great for wounds and burns. Reduces swelling and great for bee stings. Calendula is also great for healing sore eyes, stomach aches and even gum issues.

Ingredients   ## Instructions

2 tsp calendula petals

Place petals in a pot and cover with 1 cup of boiled water.

1 cup water

Let steep for 15-20 minutes and strain tea into a cup.

Pot

Add honey and lemon to taste.

Cup

Lemon

For insect bites, wounds or burns, to use as a compress, place tea soaked cloth directly on affected area. In this case, do not use the honey or lemon.

Honey

As a poultice, grind the herb and place the herb directly on affected area so that the herb oils can go directly into the wound.

Alternative Heroes

Alternative methods as mentioned above can include many elements and first among them for most people might be old reliable homemade remedies that have been passed down through generations. Products like baking soda, castor oil, onions, Epsom salt or olive oil are already in most households. Before the host of convenient chemical cure-alls available today, folks relied on the same methods their ancestors had used for centuries to heal their wounds and cure their ills. Modern studies have shown how effective those homemade healers can be with nowhere near the cost and usually no side effects.

Let's examine just a few of these household heroes that you are sure to be familiar with, although you may not know their specific health benefits.

__Apples__

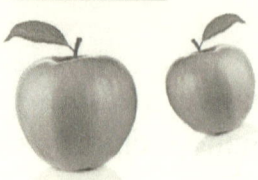

We have all heard that an apple a day keeps the doctor away, and here are a few reasons why:

- Fiber – Apples have a wealth of fiber, both soluble (prevents fats and sugar's from being absorbed into your body which helps control diabetes and cholesterol) and insoluble (absorbs cholesterol in your intestines and carries them out of your body thus preventing constipation). They are good for you whether you eat them fresh, dried, frozen, cooked or drink them as 100% apple juice.

- Studies have shown that eating apples on a regular basis can relieve or even prevent many health problems such as asthma, colds, cardiovascular disease, coronary heart disease, allergies and stroke. Keeping apples in your fridge can extend their usefulness up to six weeks.

Chamomile

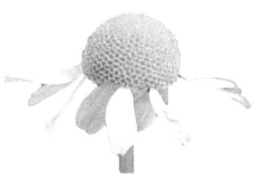

By now, nearly everyone is familiar with using chamomile as a relaxing herbal sleep aid, but did you know that there are numerous other uses which have proven effective over the years? It's been known to relieve tooth pain, upset stomach, diarrhea, anxiety and helps kill germs.

- It has powerful anti- inflammatory powers that helps reduce redness, puffiness, and irritation around your eyes. You only need to steep two tea bags in a cup of boiled water for three minutes, take them out of the water and put them in the fridge for five minutes. Then lie down and put a bag over each eye. Then relax or 15 minutes or so and you should have good results. Use this same formula for curing a stomach ache. At least three to four cups a day.

- Chamomile can be used to relieve menstrual cramps, stress related hives, even carpal tunnel syndrome, indigestion and hiccups, sore throat, toothache, sunburn and the list goes on. Research this treasure chest of herbs, you'll be glad you did.

Garlic

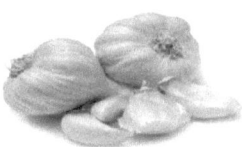

It is said that people living in garlic loving regions like the Mediterranean tend to live longer and have fewer chronic health problems than people who don't have garlic as a regular part of their diet.

- You can reduce your blood pressure by soaking ½ pound of peeled cloves in 1 quart of brandy for two weeks, shaking the mixture a few times a day, then strain it, pour it into bottles with tight fitting stoppers and drink up to 20 drops a day.

- For toothaches, quickly peel a clove, crush it, and apply it directly to the gum above or below the affected tooth.

- For sore throat, add peeled clove to two tablespoons of olive oil, heat on the stove for a minute or two. Strain it, let it cool then rub the oil on the front sides of your neck.

- You can use the same oil for earaches by putting a few drops of oil into your ear using an eye dropper. Never heat garlic in a microwave because it will kill health-giving properties.

- If you happen to lose your voice and end up with laryngitis, you may not make many new friends, but if you are willing to slice a garlic bulb in half and tuck a half into each side of your mouth, then suck on it like a lozenge.

- To fend off an approaching cold, start eating a whole clove every couple of hours. You won't be popular, but you probably will feel better.

- For constipation, eat one or two minced garlic cloves a day. Mix in milk or plain yogurt until you get relief.

- There are so many fascinating uses for this incredible herb that it would take all day to share its many possibilities and recipes for external and internal maladies.

- Just remember to consult your physician first if you are taking any kind of medication whether prescription or over the counter before you dose yourself with any garlic remedy.

Avocados

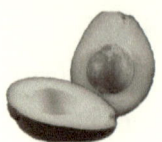

Finally this fatty plant has been widely accepted as being beneficial for both health and beauty needs. Not only do they help prevent cancer and heart disease, they also help lower cholesterol, both good and bad.

- If you need first aid for a recent cut, just break off a small piece of the fruit and rub it on the cut. It has antibiotic properties and will start working to heal the wound and ease the pain.

- If you are trying to lose weight, just mash an avocado and mix it with lemon or lime juice and you can use it as your spread or topping on toast or other dishes. You can bake with it and only use half the butter you would normally use.

- For sunburn or minor kitchen burns, just rub some of the scooped out fruit on your skin to get relief in a hurry. You can also use it to sooth the pain and itching of skin disorders like psoriasis and eczema.

- For insomnia, eat avocados on a regular basis. The potassium in this and other similar products encourages deep sleep.

- If you have been suffering from a serious illness and have lost your appetite for some time, puree an avocado and eat what you can when you can. It will provide you with loads of vitamins and minerals that you will need to build your strength and crank your system and get it to working smoothly again while it pampers your stomach.

- The natural lubrication that women enjoy tends to lessen over the years and makes intercourse unpleasant, spoiling the mood. Applying avocado oil to affected area will ease the experience and if you add in a back massage with the oil it helps you to relax and set the mood.

- Avocados have proven to be effective breath fresheners. They remove the residual aroma after eating and remove decomposing residue in your intestines which contributes to bad breath. So including avocados as a regular part of our diet could help that situation.

Lavender

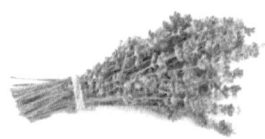

Throughout the centuries people from Cleopatra to queen Victoria have held lavender in the highest esteem for its healing and beautifying powers. Today it has universal appeal due to a myriad of uses which research has revealed.

- To keep mosquitoes away mix two parts lavender oil with one part rubbing alcohol in a plastic spray bottle and spray on your skin whenever you go outside. The bugs will stay away and you'll enjoy the scent. If you've already started to itch and swell just dab a drop of the oil on the affected area and let it sink into your skin. Repeat until you feel relief.

- Heal your burned skin quickly by spraying area with cool water and lavender oil solution.

- If you have been exposed to poison ivy, oak or sumac, you might want to try this potion. Mix three drops of lavender oil with one tablespoon of apple cider vinegar, one tablespoon of water and one half teaspoon of salt. Apply to the area with a cotton ball to ease the itch, dry out the rash and prevent infection.

- When you exercise too much and need quick relief, massage yourself with lavender oil and let the oils anti-inflammatory compounds deliver deep-down relief. Even the soothing scent will help relax you and take your mind off your discomfort.

- You might also soak your feet in a tub of hot water with five to ten drops of oil per quart of water. Let your feet soak for ten minutes or more to stimulate increased blood flow and quicker healing.

- When you feel like you can hardly breathe and your chest just won't stop hurting, you need a lavender-eucalyptus chest rub. Simply mix ten drops of lavender oil and fifteen drops of eucalyptus oil with one quarter cup of olive oil. Massage into your upper chest and cover up with a t-shirt and get in bed. It's sure to relax your muscles and kill germs while opening your breathing passages.

- Stop asthmas attacks by breathing in hot steam for quick relief. Add two tablespoons of lavender flowers for each quart of water. Boil and inhale. It should open up your passages and relax your facial muscles in very little time.

- To make the herbal tea, simply put one to two teaspoons of dried flower in boiling water and add honey and/or lemon juice to taste. It has been known to calm your nerves, heal cuts and scrapes, soothe migraines and headaches, relieves heartburn, indigestion, strengthen your gums and sweeten your breath.

__Honey__

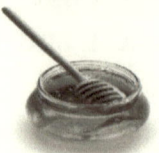

Honey is a sweet, miracle food substance produced by bees and it is a much healthier sugar alternative than refined sugar. Honey has many medicinal properties and is known to not have a shelf life. Real raw honey does not spoil.

- If you suffer from acid indigestion you need only take one to three teaspoons of honey for quick relief.

- An old fashioned but effective remedy for arthritis is as simple as mixing one teaspoon of honey with one teaspoon of apple cider vinegar. Take this every morning and every evening for great relief.

- For bee sting, just remove the stinger and put a dab of honey on the spot for quick relief.

- For cuts and scrapes, wash the wound and spread honey over the area. It blocks infection causing microorganisms and forms a natural bandage that promotes healing.

- To avoid getting a hangover, before you start drinking, eat a piece of toast or a few crackers with a generous amount of honey on it. If you forget, you should still eat some after you stop drinking to avoid a serious hangover.

- To improve your ability to go to sleep quickly, mix one teaspoon of honey in a glass of warm milk or lukewarm water and drink it all to drift off to sleep quickly.

- To lose weight, mix two teaspoons of honey in a glass of water half an hour before each meal. This will naturally suppress your appetite so you won't be tempted to overeat.

- To get relief from a serious hacking cough, mix a full cup of honey with one half cup of olive oil and four tablespoons of fresh-squeezed lemon juice. Heat on low for five minutes, stir for two minutes, pour in a tight-fitting jar and keep at room temperature. Take one teaspoon every two hours as needed.

- For constipation, mix a tablespoon or two in a glass of warm water and drink.

Herbal Contraindications

Aloe Vera – Children under 12 years old, pregnant or lactating women and people with bowel issues or on medication should consult their doctors before ingesting Aloe Vera. The plant is known to have negative effects in these cases.

Basil – Considered safe for all, even pregnant women when taken in capsules or used in foods in small amounts. Basil also known to be safe for children in small amounts. It is a great herb known to have many medicinal and healing properties and is a great culinary flavor in many dishes.

Burdock – Avoid during pregnancy and lactation. May cause allergic reactions.

Cayenne Pepper – Cayenne pepper could interfere with medications. Pregnant or lactating women should not consume cayenne pepper.

Calendula – There are no recorded side effects for using this herb. However, pregnant and lactating women should consult with their physicians before using this herb.

Chamomile – Should not be used by pregnant or lactating women or people who are allergic to ragweed pollens.

Chickweed – There are no recorded side effects or cautions with this plant. It's loaded with the vitamins and minerals that the body needs.

Cinnamon – Pregnant women should consult their physicians before using cinnamon because it can cause contractions. People with hypersensitivity to cinnamon should use with caution. No other contraindications identified.

Dandelion – Safe for pregnant women when eaten as a food. However, everyone should consult their doctors before taking dandelion to ensure safe dosages when taken as a supplement or dosages above those found in foods.

Echinacea - Those with compromised immune systems should steer clear of echinacea. It can cause allergic reactions in some people and those with asthma should not take this herb. Echinacea doesn't mix well with medicines for the immune system. Pregnant and lactating women should consult with their physician before using this herb.

Elder (Elderberry) – People with diabetes should not use elderberry. Do not consume elder products two weeks before or after surgery. The elder plant is not safe for pregnant or lactating women.

Ginger – Ginger is very strong and can interact with certain medications causing negative side effects. Always consult with your doctor before giving ginger to children. Pregnant and lactating women should consult with their doctors or just stay away from using ginger until after lactation periods.

Garlic – Garlic is generally regarded as safe. However, people with stomach ulcers, digestive issues or bleeding disorders should not use garlic. Lactating women should not use garlic as it can pass into the breast milk and make the child sick. Garlic is not a recommended supplement for children. Garlic can weaken the effect of birth control pills. Consult with your doctor about ways to avoid pregnancy if you're on garlic supplements or eat a lot of garlic.

Hawthorn – The Hawthorne plant is general regarded as safe and has no known recorded side effects.

Lavender – Not recommended for internal use for pregnant and lactating women. Lavender taken internally can have a negative interaction with certain medications. Always consult your physician before internal use.

Lemon Balm – Not for pregnant and lactating women. Lemon balm should not be consumed or used by people with hypothyroid issues. Always consult with your physician first before using this herb internally.

Liquorice – Not for pregnant or lactating women. Liquorice can increase blood pressure and since it has laxative effects on many people, it can expel much needed potassium from the body which is not good for pregnant women, diabetics or anyone suffering from low potassium levels or high blood pressure. Do not exceed the recommended daily amount.

Marshmallow – Diabetics should not take Marshmallow since it is known to interfere with blood sugar levels. Lactating and pregnant women should consult with their physicians before consuming this herb. Anyone facing a surgery should stop taking marshmallow two weeks before and two weeks after surgery.

Nettle – Can cause uterine contractions in pregnant women. Not recommended at all for pregnant and lactating mothers. Nettle increases urine flow so if there's a history of fluid retention, Nettle is not considered a safe herb to take without first consulting with your physician.

Plantain – Not for pregnant or lactating mothers. Plantain can trigger allergic reactions. People using lithium or carbamazepine should consult with their doctors before using or consuming this product.

Red Clover – For those with hormone sensitive issues such as breast cancer should not use Red Clover. Pregnant and lactating mothers should consult with their doctors before using this herb. It is generally regarded as safe when consuming by mouth in small quantities. Red Clover may reduce blood clotting and should not be taken two weeks before or two weeks after surgery.

Rosemary – Use caution when taking large amounts of Rosemary by mouth. Can cause vomiting, uterine bleeding, kidney irritation and allergic reactions. Pregnant and lactating mothers should avoid Rosemary unless approved by a physician.

Sage – Generally regarded as safe for all. Pregnant women should consult with their physicians before using any herb.

Peppermint – No known negative side effects. It is considered non-toxic and a non-irritant.

Spearmint – No known negative side effects. It is considered non-toxic and a non-irritant.

St. John's Wort – People with severe depression or who are taking antidepressants, blood thinners and other mind altering drugs should not use St. John's Wort. St. John's Wort might also cause severe reactions to sun exposure.

Thyme – This herb has no recorded side effects or cautions. However, pregnant and lactating women should always consult with their physicians before taking herbs.

Turmeric – This plant has no known recorded side-effects. However, pregnant and lactating women should always consult with their physicians before taking herbs.

Valerian – Safe for short term use but may cause mild side effects such as headache, uneasiness, dizziness, and even insomnia. Do not use Valerian while operating heavy machinery. Pregnant and lactating women should always consult with their physicians before using this herb.

Yarrow – Pregnant women should not use this herb as it could cause miscarriage. Avoid using if you're taking blood thinning medications like Warfarin, Lithium, acid-reducing medications and high blood pressure medications. This herb is like safe when taken by mouth in small amounts or amounts commonly found in food. This herb could increase urination and cause dizziness. Do not use on children. Always consult your physician before using this herb.

To make this guide more useful as a functioning reference I have included this list of contraindicators that are vital to beginning your journey through nature's most beneficial gifts-herbs. This by no means should replace your own personal research but it will certainly compliment and enhance it.

Why herbs? Herbs are used to stimulate the body's self-healing powers and remove the underlying cause of illness. Then the herbs are used to nourish and tone all the organs and systems of the body from the inside out. However, prior to using herbs, it's wise to do a total body flush of the colon, lymph systems and cleansing of the blood to have the desired effect of the herbs to do their jobs. Research herbal cleanses on the web and you will find a number of choices to clean your system. I used Dr. Sebi products at: www.drsebiproducts.com. Dr. Sebi is a well-known master herbalist whose products I have used for years.

Physicians and folk healers have relied on medicinal plants since ancient times. Even today researchers are searching the plant for more healing herbs. In fact, herbal medicine is a precursor of model pharmacology and about one fourth of all prescription medicines come from herbs and other plants. Today, physicians and researchers are taking a new look at traditional herbal remedies.

At one time or another, every society has relied upon the healing power of herbs to treat illness, and in some, herbal medicine still prevails. The more we study herbal life and merge them with conventional applications, the more our quality of life will improve as God has intended for it to be.

Remedies Index

Page

Arterial Plaque	30
Arthritis	31
Bladder (Urinary Tract)	29
Bloating	27
Blood Cleansing	24, 38
Breath (Halitosis)	24, 38
Bronchitis	28
Cholesterol	30, 36
Colds and Flu	23, 30, 34, 35, 37
Constipation	30
Diarrhea	25, 26, 38
Digestion/Indigestion	25, 26, 33, 36, 38, 40
Diuretic	39
Fatigue	23
Flatulence (Gas)	26, 27
Gum Health	29, 40
Headache	25, 26, 30
Herpes (Mouth Sores)	28, 31
Hot Flashes	24, 30

Remedies Index (cont.)

	Page
Inflammation & Pain	31, 36
Kidney Issues	27, 30
Menopause	24, 27, 30
Menstrual Cramps	26, 27, 30
Nausea	26
Sore Throat	28
Stress and Concentration	23, 24, 25, 28, 30, 32
Toothache	29
Tuberculosis	28
Ulcers	30
Wounds	28, 30, 38, 39

www.ingramcontent.com/pod-product-compliance
Lightning Source LLC
Chambersburg PA
CBHW020401290526
45785CB00005B/2388